SIMPLE WAYS TO RELAX

mind, body & soul

Barbara L. Heller

*The mission of Storey Publishing is to serve our customers
by publishing practical information that encourages personal independence
in harmony with the environment.*

Edited by Deborah Balmuth and Karen Levy
Cover design by Wendy Palitz
Cover background illustrations by Alexandra Eckhardt
Cover image art © Juliette Borda
Text design and production by Susan Bernier

The text of this book was excerpted from *365 Ways to Relax Mind, Body & Soul* (Storey, 2000).

Printed in the United States by Lake Book
10 9 8 7 6 5 4 3 2

ISBN 1-58017-895-2

Introduction

Are you stressed-out from juggling work, family, and personal activities? Feeling frazzled by excessive demands and information overload? If so, you are not alone. More than 20 million Americans suffer from stress-related illnesses. Many more are simply tired from the frenzied pace of modern life.

As a psychotherapist and educator for the past two decades, I have listened to clients, students, colleagues, and friends bemoan their increasing levels of stress, illness, and tension. And, of course, I have experienced my own challenges and anxieties. I have discovered that what we have in common is the need to develop better ways to respond to tension, loss, and frustration. We need to make more graceful transitions between our various roles and responsibilities, find new ways to wind down and replenish ourselves, and learn how to lighten up and appreciate our daily lives!

Most of us have not been taught how to relax. But relaxation is an acquired skill — one that you can learn. True relaxation creates a calm center to return to after stressful events and helps you feel renewed any time of the day. Relaxation also provides a peaceful counterpoint to positive stimulation. Releasing tension improves your immunity and heightens your creativity, effectiveness, intuition, and joy.

The benefits of relaxation are cumulative. Today, the gains may seem small, but, over time, you will be repaid with great riches. As you learn how to relax, you'll stop focusing primarily on your destination and you'll more fully enjoy the steps you take on your daily journey. The ripples will be far-reaching, affecting your family, work-place, and larger community. Relaxation will help you thrive, not just survive.

This little book offers you a broad range of relaxation techniques and soothing remedies and recipes. Many of the simple, practical tips you can try right now. Others require some planning and aim to create long-term solutions to stress. Start by choosing a couple of tips and incorporating them into your usual routine for five minutes a day. Build on your success. In the end, you will gain a healthier body, a calmer mind, and a more peaceful spirit.

Barbara L. Heller, M.S.W.

Express your creativity. All you need is a "little kid" coloring book with old favorite cartoon characters, an extra large box of crayons, and no artistic standards. And don't be afraid to color outside the lines!

Clean out the clutter. Mental clutter may keep you from falling asleep, but physical clutter can affect you as well. Take some time this week to clean up the piles of clothes, stacks of magazines, or numerous knickknacks that are cluttering your bedroom. A simplified environment serves as a natural sedative.

"Finish each day and be done with it. You have done what you could. Tomorrow is a new day; begin it well and serenely and with too high a spirit to be encumbered with your old nonsense."

—Ralph Waldo Emerson

Practice the cat stretch. This wonderful yoga stretch, which increases flexibility and improves breathing, gets its inspiration from the sensual, expansive curls of a cat.

1. Get down on all fours with your hands directly under your shoulders and your knees right under your hips (the "table position").

2. Breathe out, slowly rounding your back up and gently dropping your chin to your chest. Continue to breathe and hold the position for a count of 5.

3. Breathe in, raising your head and slowly uncurling so that your back is slightly arched and you are looking straight ahead. Hold for a count of 5.

4. Repeat 5 times. Purr-fect!

Let your cares float away during a day on the water. Cruise the currents in a small, nonmotorized boat. Canoeing is calming, and sailing is serene.

Carry an umbrella. Being prepared minimizes stress. So purchase a few small, fold-up umbrellas. Leave one in your car, another in your attaché or at the office. Then you'll never worry about getting caught in the rain.

Eat dessert first. The strawberries are ripe and the short-cake is made. Why wait?

Get out those old 33 rpm records. A musical friend assures me that records have been scientifically proven to provide a more soothing sound to the ear than CDs and cassettes. Remember Johnny Mathis, Judy Collins, the Beatles? Turn on the record player and groove to your old favorites.

"A rich world of wonder awaits."

—Carl Sagan

Are you constantly looking at your watch while waiting in line at the supermarket? Are you impatient before an appointment or until your children's lessons are finished? Treat yourself to a "waiting enhancer." Carry a favorite magazine or paperback book in your bag to while away the time pleasantly.

Let the morning sun shine on you. Bright natural light early in the day enhances your body's internal rhythms and helps you sleep better at night.

Take a jog or an aerobics class. More than 70 percent of people say that they don't work out because they are too tired, but what they may not know is that exercise is a great stress reliever. If you break the fatigue–inactivity cycle, you will be rewarded with relaxation.

After a tiring day, soothe those tight muscles by filling the bathtub with 2 cups of Epsom salts and hot water (stimulating, but not scalding). Sink into the tub and lounge with a towel or bath pillow behind your head. When the water begins to cool, stand up and turn on the shower. Rinse off with a blast of cold water, then end with a warming stream.

Essential oils are highly concentrated essences derived from plants and flowers. Relax with the sedating scents of lavender, lemon balm, Roman chamomile, neroli, ylang ylang, and clary sage.

Who wants to cook when it's hot? Partnered with bakery-bought bread, cold soups are simple and satisfying summer fare. Try chilled gazpacho, a spicy Spanish vegetable soup prepared in a blender.

Postpone procrastination. We often put off unpleasant tasks. We stall because we are afraid of making decisions or mistakes. This just prolongs our tension and discomfort. Figure out the reasons for your procrastination. Then, don't delay. Do it now!

Write your own horoscope. Don't you sometimes wish the overgeneralized newspaper horoscopes were right? Make believe. "Grab the brass ring and do what you have wanted to do for a long time," or "The stars are right for romance." Live today with that possibility.

"If you take your time and keep your wits about you, you can cultivate a wholesome and artful spiritual life that nourishes the whole self — one that will help you enjoy the world and perhaps even save it."

—Elizabeth Lesser

Schedule a worry session. If you honor your concerns for a focused half-hour, you may eliminate being plagued by worries throughout the day. Reserve a quiet time and place to sit and worry. Then, when you feel distressed outside of the specified time, say to yourself, "Don't worry now. You have plenty of time to worry later."

"There will be time enough to do it all. But not all at once."

—Wayne Sotile

What does relaxation mean to you? How do you feel when you are relaxed? Write a list of relaxing words on an index card and keep it at your desk as a reminder. Here are some to start you off — calm, peaceful, quiet, blissful, still, comfortable, mellow, tranquil, warm, cozy, hushed, luxurious, slow, easy, refreshed.

Lessen your holiday stress by limiting gifts to a pre-planned amount. Enhance the spiritual meaning of the season while eliminating credit card debt.

Give yourself a hand . . . a hand massage, that is. Using the thumb and index finger of your left hand, squeeze each finger on your right hand, one by one. Make rolling movements from your knuckles to your fingertips. Gently pull each finger, then switch hands.

What song best reflects your personal goals? What piece of music could help you maintain your calm center during a hectic day? Try humming your favorite tune before a dreaded meeting or singing your chosen song in the shower or car. Who knows? Soon you may hear those around you tapping to your beat.

Play some peaceful "mind movies." Visualization engages your calm, creative center. Imagine a peaceful lake. Paint a picture with all of your senses. See the water's shimmering ripples, feel the gentle breeze, hear the call of the loons, and smell the fresh air. Picture yourself sitting there alone, breathing slowly and enjoying the tranquillity of the outdoors. Take this sense of serenity with you as you continue with your day.

Plan a celebration. Imagine a silly but special one. If you're the dramatic type, celebrate the Academy Awards, either by yourself or with a couple of close friends. Don your fanciest clothes and serve an elegantly simple spread. Smoked oysters, anyone? If you love Goofy and the rest of the Disney gang, make sure that they are represented at your birthday celebrations. What will you wear and what specialties will you serve?

Enjoy a Magical Drink

To many New Yorkers, egg creams are more than drinks — they evoke the wonder of childhood, and sipping one brings back memories of slower days. Actually, egg creams don't contain any eggs or cream and are only a fancy fizzed version of chocolate milk! Makes 1 serving.

   3 tablespoons chocolate syrup
   ⅓ cup ice-cold milk
   ⅔ cup seltzer

1. Pour the chocolate syrup into a tall glass.
2. Add the milk and stir.
3. Fill the rest of the glass with the seltzer while stirring. You've got it right when the top third of the glass is thickly foamed.

"You must learn to be still in the midst of activity and to be vibrantly alive in repose."

—Indira Gandhi

Food of the gods. Recent studies suggest that there is no reason to feel guilty about your craving for chocolate. A dietary source of magnesium, chocolate contains antioxidants and heart-healthy compounds. Even if it weren't so good for you, a delicious chocolate treat is relaxing.

Valerian is the premier herb to treat insomnia and stress. German studies have proven its benefits as a relaxant without sedative side effects. When valerian is paired with the more pleasant-tasting lemon balm, its strong odor is masked while its relaxing qualities are enhanced. Try this combination in liquid extracts or capsules.

Start lunch with a bowl of soup. Soup sipping encourages slower meals. Studies show that people who begin their meals with soup consume fewer calories.

Child's pose. This gentle reclining yoga position is relaxing and will help you sleep better.

1. Kneel on the floor. Spread your knees shoulder-width apart while keeping your feet together. Lower your buttocks onto your heels.
2. Bend forward. Lower your chest to your knees.
3. Place your head on the floor with your face turned to one side or with your forehead resting on the ground.
4. Rest for a few minutes with your arms by your sides and your palms up. Breathe slowly and deeply.

Letting go of an old regret or shameful memory is often difficult but always liberating. What would help you heal? How can you shed the weight of a past transgression? Write about it in your journal. Or find a truly sympathetic person to share your secret with — a friend, support group member, or counselor.

Enjoy a trashy novel. Don't be embarrassed — reading sappy, silly, or simple books is a wonderful form of no-stress entertainment. So cruise over to the library or bookstore and stock up! Books with "no redeeming value" are golden for lying on the couch on a cold winter's day or for packing in your beach bag for a summer idyll.

Lavender Lullaby

It's easy and relaxing to make and use bath salts at home.

⅓ cup baking soda   ⅓ cup sea salt
⅓ cup Epsom salts   10 drops lavender essential oil

1. In a nonporous bowl, combine the baking soda, Epsom salts, and sea salt. Add the lavender essential oil.
2. Cover mixture with a cotton cloth; leave to dry overnight.
3. In the morning, stir the mixture to break up any chunks. Store it in a pretty bottle or tin.

To use, pour ½ cup of the salts into the tub as it is filling with warm water.

Remember. Relive pleasant memories. Save some favorite cards and letters to reread while sipping a cup of tea. Appreciate the connections and comfort of your larger community.

*"**Moving toward an inwardly simple life** is not about deprivation or denying ourselves the things we want. It's about getting rid of the things that no longer contribute to the fullness of our lives. It's about creating balance between our inner and outer lives."*

—Elaine St. James

At the first sign of spring, take a hike in the woods, stroll along the shore of a lake, sit in a sunny garden, or take a walk on the beach. Seasonal relaxation engages the senses. Where can you go to renew your connection with the healing power of the earth?

Relaxation is contagious. Spend time with calm companions.

Develop a new way of seeing. A creative teacher used this technique to help his students gain a new visual perspective. Add one drop of red ink to a full glass of water and you might see an angel, rubies, or a favorite relative. Stop, look around you, and change one small detail. The new things you observe may surprise you.

Turn off the television. The majority of American families spend more time watching television every day than they do speaking to each other. If you're not ready to eliminate all television time, try to cut your viewing by half. Use the extra time to chat with family members or just enjoy the newfound silence.

Before video games and computers, folks relaxed together around the game board. Dust off those old favorites hiding in the back of the cabinet or purchase new ones for some Friday evening fun.

Choose a comforting commuting companion. Garrison Keillor produces the Writer's Almanac, a quirky five-minute morning show on National Public Radio. Are country songs more to your liking? How about a local talk-show personality who makes you laugh? Invite someone along on your morning drive.

Humor is healing, and a night of laughter is good for the soul. Watch *I Love Lucy* reruns and videotapes of original funny favorites, such as Laurel and Hardy or Charlie Chaplin.

Go fly a kite. Find relaxing fun in a windy field where you can feel the breeze and the freedom of flight.

Feeling anxious and out-of-sorts? Come back to yourself with this breathing exercise.

1. Place the index and middle fingers of your left hand horizontally across your chin and press gently.
2. At the same time, place the index and middle fingers of your right hand 2 inches below your navel and press.
3. Drop your shoulders and take four deep breaths. (This can also help stop a case of the hiccups.)

You don't have to tiptoe through the tulips to appreciate the many different textures under your feet. Indoor rugs, outdoor grass, and cool paving stones can soothe your sole.

Don't be a victim of your hairdo! Consult with a talented hairstylist and choose a versatile wash-and-wear style that looks attractive and lessens morning primp time. Bring magazine pictures to the salon to showcase the right look.

Reduce road rage. Anticipate traffic jams and the driving habits of other people. When possible, adjust your travel time to eliminate rush hour. Don't distract yourself by talking on a cellular phone; instead, calm down by listening to Sylvia Boorstein's *Road Sage* on audio cassette.

Live with a poem for a week. Recite it daily. Reflect on the questions and meanings your chosen poem inspires. Poet Mary Oliver provides interesting food for thought when she asks, "What is it you plan to do with your one wild and precious life?"

Don't carry the weight of the world; shrug it off! Shoulder shrugs are easy stretches that release tension from your upper body. You can do them while either sitting or standing.

1. Inhale and tighten your shoulders, pulling them up toward your ears.
2. Exhale and gently release.
3. Repeat three times.
4. Enjoy your relaxed shoulders!

Rescue Remedy, a flower essence developed by Dr. Edward Bach in the 1930s, is a calming and stabilizing treatment for stress and trauma. This five-flower formula is nontoxic, nonaddictive, and free from any known side effects. Take it in small doses throughout a stressful day. Rescue Remedy is available at health food stores and natural pharmacies.

Relaxing Massage Oil

It's easy to make your own massage oil for treating tense muscles.

    4 teaspoons sweet almond oil
    5 drops lavender essential oil
    5 drops sandalwood essential oil

1. Combine the ingredients.
2. Apply the oil blend to tense muscles with long flowing strokes.

Plan a personal pampering party. Turn off the phone, sift through a pile of magazines, give yourself a manicure, write a letter, loll in the bath, and plan your next creative endeavor.

Chew slowly. Be conscious of each portion of food you put in your mouth and put your fork down in between bites.

Swan stretch. This stretch helps release chronic tension and gracefully lengthens your neck.

1. Sit in a cross-legged position on the floor with your back straight and your hands resting on your thighs.
2. Stretch your right arm out to the side and touch the floor with your right hand.
3. Inhale and stretch your head to the left. Don't lean forward. Feel the stretch from your head to your hands.
4. Exhale and release any tension into the ground through your fingers.
5. Inhale and straighten your head while returning your right hand to your thigh.
6. Repeat on the other side.

"If trying harder doesn't work, try softer."

—Lily Tomlin

Describe the most pleasant and relaxing time you've ever experienced. Were you at home, on vacation, at a spa, or on a retreat? Were you alone or with others? What were you wearing and what did you eat? Do one small thing today that reminds you of that peaceful time.

Be an herbal copycat with catnip. Catnip-stuffed toys may stimulate your feline, but the herb has the opposite effect on people. Catnip, a tasty and easy-to-grow cousin of mint, makes a mild sedative tea.

Designate today as your personal aroma day. Switch gears by stretching your sense of smell. Ask yourself these three questions: Which scents delight me? Which aromas relax me? What might I smell today?

Cultivate a heart of stillness. Find a deep sense of inner peace by recommitting to your house of worship or finding a new spiritual home through a church group or personal prayer.

Seek the secrets of silence. Meditation teaches us how to quiet our overactive brains and experience a sense of serenity. Books, tapes, and classes can help you learn this potent method of self-observation.

Pop singer Paul Simon once crooned, "Everyone loves the sound of a train in the distance." Listen to the rhythmic clacking of a train and the whistle marking its approach. You can't hurry the train. Just notice it and breathe slowly until its music fades away.

When you are "breathless" in anticipation or "frozen with fear," your breathing becomes shallow. Alleviate your anxiety by consciously altering the rhythm and depth of your breathing. Put one hand on your chest and the other on your abdomen. Create a quiet wave between your chest and belly by slowing and deepening your breath.

Pace yourself for a peaceful day. Be aware of the time of day when you are most alert. Schedule that time to tackle creative or difficult tasks. Allot languid times for easier activities.

Simmer a small amount of cloves, cinnamon, and orange peel in two cups of water on top of the stove. The soothing fragrance will fill your home.

Nose alphabets. Here's a quick way to ease tense neck muscles.

1. Sit up straight with your head forward and your shoulders relaxed.

2. Move your nose in small, smooth movements to trace the alphabet in the air — half-inch capital letters are best.

You may get some strange looks, but when others find out about this simple relaxing exercise, they may join you.

"Beauty of style and harmony and grace and good rhythm depend on simplicity."

—Plato

Travel light. Lugging heavy and bulky luggage is stressful. Instead, choose a few mix-and-match outfits and pack a small rolling valise and a matching carry-on bag.

Lose those shoes and loosen your tie. Choreograph your own calm by moving to a slow tempo. Five minutes on your feet followed by five minutes of sitting still is a great stress reducer.

Don't stifle that sigh. As renowned yoga instructor Lillias Folan observed, "We have too many unsighed sighs inside of us." Let yours out. An audible exhalation acknowledges and releases tension.

Give yourself a time cushion. Dreaded deadlines increase stress. For any pending project, pencil in your planner a personal deadline that is days or weeks before the actual deadline. If the computer crashes or you get a cold, you'll have the relief of extra time.

Don't bring work home. Make a transition at your front door. Purge the cares of the day by paring down overly practical and technological details. Don't allow your bedroom to do double duty as a mini-office. Put your desk and computer in another room or screen them from view with a pretty room divider.

The lion pose. Roars are relaxing. Let one out while practicing the Lion Pose, a tension-relieving yoga position.

1. Sit quietly with your eyes closed. Inhale through your nose.
2. Open your mouth wide and stick out your tongue. Stretch it down toward your chin.
3. Stretch your eyes into a wide stare; look up.
4. Let out a roar as you loudly exhale.
5. Close your mouth and relax your eyes.
6. Repeat.

Sitting at the computer for hours encourages slouching and muscle cramps. To release tension, take short breaks and change your position hourly. Push your chair back and close your eyes or stand up and stretch.

Cleaning out your closets lessens the amount you have to organize, clean, and repair. And that frees up time to relax.

Forget "No pain, no gain." Instead, try smooth stretching movements. Resist the tendency to bounce or push past discomfort. Breathe deeply while gently loosening. Repeat similar movements on both sides of your body.

Relaxation. How many words can you make with the letters from the word relaxation?

Coffee-table books cure cabin fever. They can transport you to the tropics during the winter or take you someplace cool and breezy when it's hot and humid outside. Try oversized library books full of photos for inspiration. Or browse through *National Geographic* and travel magazines.

Who seems to live the calm, balanced life that you crave? Ask the people you admire how they do it. You may be surprised by their challenges and helped by their resources, tools, and ideas.

Brush your hair. Tradition recommends 100 strokes nightly, but gently brushing your hair without counting may be more relaxing. To encourage healthy hair growth and enhance thickness, add 1 or 2 drops of rosemary essential oil to your hairbrush.

Keep your hands busy and the rest of you will slow down. Devote 15 minutes daily to needlework. Stitch a serene scene preprinted on canvas. Starter kits are available at craft stores. To prolong the relaxation benefits, display the finished piece in your work area.

Serve yourself a glass of ice-cold lemonade and sip it through a straw.

Find an antidote for the "Arsenic Hour," the stressful period right before dinner. Tame this tense time with an array of preplanned activities and guidelines for the kids. Have on hand some simple nutritious snacks, such as carrot and celery sticks or cheese and crackers. Limit telephone, television, and computer use and play some quiet background music instead.

Invite your family or friends to a movie marathon — at home. Combine some classics with new releases. Pass the popcorn.

Just say NO. Overloaded with too many tasks, we still often agree to one more responsibility. This month pass on all requests for your participation. Clearing the decks will help you decide what is most important to you. And remember, next month when you are calm and centered, you can agree to serve on that committee.

Hold that pose. Stop and become aware of your posture. Are you slumped in your chair? Feeling tense or tight? If so, don't quickly change positions. Exhale fully and gently exaggerate your stance. Then inhale and slowly straighten.

Prolonged desk work causes tight shoulders and upper arms. Take a minibreak and rub the stress away with a self-massage.

1. Place your left hand on your right shoulder.
2. Gently knead the muscles between your neck and arm.
3. Squeeze. Hold for a few seconds, then release.
4. Continue to gently squeeze and rub along your shoulder and upper arm.
5. Repeat on your left side.

When your hands are overused and underappreciated, they're at risk for strain injuries. Be sure to take breaks from typing and other tasks that require repetitive hand movements. Wiggle your fingers, then stretch them wide apart. Make a fist with your whole hand and release it. Then gently shake the tension out of your hands.

White knuckles on the wheel and a lead foot on the pedal may get you there a bit faster — but you'll also be frazzled. Getting to work shouldn't be a race. Allow 5 to 10 extra minutes for your morning drive.

Listen for the sounds of the seasons. Autumn is marked by honking geese announcing their departure for warmer climes; the red robin's morning song signals spring. Wherever you live, whether city, suburb, or countryside, notice how nature's music changes throughout the year.

As the song goes, "Summertime and the living is easy." That's when meal preparation should be quick and uncomplicated. Have a salad for supper on a summer's eve. Eat on the porch or picnic in the park.

Turn off the alarm clock. If you need an alarm to wake up, you are probably sleep deprived. This weekend, catch up on needed rest and wake up naturally.

Tame tension headaches with this simple technique.
1. Place your index and middle fingers of both hands at the outer edges of your eyebrows and on the indentations at your temples.
2. Rub in small circular movements.
3. Increase the pressure and hold for a count of 2.
4. Release; repeat as necessary.

Simplify holiday gift giving. Instead of searching for the perfect gift, choose a theme, such as books or kitchen supplies, and buy similar presents for everyone on your list.

When we're tired and tense, we often choose time-wasting activities that don't rejuvenate us. Replace Web surfing with listening to a tape of soothing music or doing a half-hour of yoga. Free up your free time for some really relaxing activities.

Share the work and savor the leisure time. Make sure that everyone on your home team is responsible for his or her own area. Even young children can do simple chores. Older family members can do their own laundry, and dinner preparation can be rotated.

*"**Be willing to live** in between right and wrong. The ego needs and desperately wants to be right and make others wrong. In between right and wrong is a soft, messy, laughing place where it doesn't matter."*

—SARK

Elementary school teachers have the right idea when they tell their classes how best to relax. It works for adults, too! Push your chair back. Lean forward from your waist. Rest your forehead on your folded arms on your desk. Your productivity and creativity will get a jump start with a five-minute break.

Save some seashells from the beach. Bring them home and relive the serenity of the seashore with this simple meditation.

1. Place a seashell in front of you. Sit quietly and pay attention to your breathing.
2. Gaze at the shell. Move your eyes around its curves.
3. Sense the shell without describing it. When words or judgments pop up, just let them pass.
4. Sit like this for 5 to 10 minutes before you return to other activities.

Designate today as your personal sight day. Release your thoughts and worries by stretching your sense of sight. Ask yourself these three questions: Which sights delight me? Which sights relax me? What might I see today?

Vanilla's deep, sweet scent summons a sense of calm. Light a vanilla-scented candle, moisturize with a vanilla lotion, or add a dash of pure vanilla extract to your cup of decaffeinated coffee.

Play with clay. Get your hands dirty; pottery making is an acceptable way to make a mess. Squeezing and molding clay releases tension. You can make functional or abstract pieces right at your kitchen table with a variety of products that you can bake or dry naturally. Or sign up for a beginner's pottery class.

Get out of your chair and do the twist. Stand face forward with your feet comfortably apart. Bend your knees slightly. Swing your arms backward and forward across your body several times. With or without music, this tempo will help you release tension.

Crystals are beautiful and have various healing potentials. Amethyst is calming and soothing; quartz is balancing. Display the crystals in your bedroom, family room, or meditation area.

The average adult needs seven to nine hours of sleep a night to function well. Most Americans get only six hours or less. Insufficient sleep is both physically and psychologically stressful. An extra 45 minutes of sleep can increase your immunity and improve your overall well-being.

Tame your restless "monkey mind" with a mantra, a syllable or word silently repeated or softly spoken during meditation. Intoning "peace," "relax," "om," or "one" will slow down your overactive mind.

Take a slow shower. Showers are mistakenly viewed as the stimulating sibling of the sedative bath. But steamy showers can be sensual and relaxing. Linger and let the water massage your tense muscles.

After a tiring day, ensure a foundation of rest. Indulge in comfortable bedding, such as a downy comforter and a large mattress. Sink into the caresses of a feather bed. Buy the softest sheets you can afford. Choose cool, all-cotton sheets in summer and try a set of flannel sheets to keep you warm in winter. Sleep in your own cradle of comfort.

Kava kava is an ancient ceremonial and medicinal herb from the South Pacific islands. It's a wonderful remedy for mild to moderate anxiety. Health food stores and natural pharmacies stock capsules and extracts. Follow the label directions.

Sleepy Time Bath Bags

Try this recipe for a soothing, sleep-inducing bath. Makes 6 bath bags.

1 cup dried chamomile flowers
1 cup dried lavender flowers
½ cup dried hops
½ cup dried rose petals

1. Combine the ingredients.
2. Pour ½ cup of the mixture into small cotton or muslin drawstring bags. When running the bath, loop the drawstring over the faucet so the water runs through the bag as the tub fills.

Acupressure points. A handy way to relieve general aches and pains is to massage the pressure point on each palm.

1. Use the thumb and index finger of one hand to squeeze the soft tissue between the thumb and index finger of the other hand.
2. Press, hold for a count of 3, and release.
3. Repeat two times on each hand.

Avoid alcoholic beverages before bedtime. Although alcohol may help you doze off, its stimulant qualities disrupt deep sleep. Substitute an evening cup of warm milk or herbal tea for a hot toddy.

If you have problems sleeping, reset your body clock by keeping to a curfew. Go to bed at the same time every night and get up at the same time every morning.

Convert a cozy corner or empty room into a place to meditate. Choose a comfortable chair or cushion to sit on. Add a CD player for soft music. Decorate the walls and floor with peaceful artwork. For privacy, separate the area from the rest of the house with gently flowing curtains or a screen.

Have a spa-rty. This is the adult version of a slumber party with a theme. Ask each guest to bring supplies for a spa treatment, such as hair conditioners, facials, and manicures. Share secrets while shampooing each other's hair.

Design a bedtime ritual. Reserve the last hour before bed for soaking in the bath, reading in a comfortable chair, and listening to instrumental music. This restful routine will help you release the day's concerns.

A sleep survey found that those who walked at least six blocks a day at a normal pace were one-third less likely to have trouble sleeping than nonwalkers. Those who walked faster decreased their risk of sleep disorders by 50 percent. If you are enlisting exercise as a sleep aid, afternoon workouts have the most benefit; don't exercise within three to five hours of bedtime.

"Don't just do something. *Sit there.*"

—Sylvia Boorstein

Transform your bedroom into a restful sanctuary. Reserve this room for sleeping, reflecting, and romancing. Surround yourself with dreamlike images. Eliminate flashy or distracting artwork, bedding, wall coverings, and window treatments. View only gentle beauty from your bed. This will enhance your mood and the quality of your sleep.

Listen closely: The signs of serenity are often more subtle than the symptoms of stress.

Muscle relaxation and anxiety are incompatible. As you contract and release your muscles, you release stress.

1. Flex your left foot, then point your toes. Don't strain; continue to breathe slowly and deeply.
2. Hold for 5 seconds and then release. Repeat with your right foot.
3. Contract and release your calf, knee, and thigh muscles. Continue to tense, hold, and release. Alternate sides of your body.
4. Contract and release your groin and stomach area, your back, and your arms and hands.
5. Proceed to your neck, face, and head.
6. Rub your hands together and gently place your warm palms over your eyes.

Create a relaxation haven. Keep a file of magazine pictures of serene bedrooms. Note the similarities in colors, shapes, and textures of rooms that appeal to you. Add some of these relaxing touches to your own bedroom.

Make a sour face . . . it won't stay that way. Tightening and releasing facial muscles is relaxing and can keep tension headaches in check. Squeeze your eyes tight, scrunch your nose, and pucker your lips as if you're eating a sour lemon. Take a deep breath and release.

Desperately seeking serenity in all the wrong places? Ditch the Friday evening happy hour. Instead, take an end-of-the-week retreat. Order some healthy take-out food, pick up a good book or video, and get to bed early.

This simple visualization exercise can help you release your cares and worries. Sit quietly and close your eyes. Picture a basket on your lap. Name your burdensome concerns, one by one, as you put them into the container. Imagine walking to a stream and pouring the basket's contents into the rushing water. Watch your worries float away. And when you return to the real world, remember that the flowing water continues to carry your cares and troubles downstream.

"We embark upon the creation *of a peaceful lifestyle by recognizing the need, daily, to cleanse our minds just as we cleanse our bodies. Through morning prayers and meditation, we embark upon the day spiritually prepared. Without this preparation, we enter the day with yesterday's anxieties — our own and those of millions of others."*

—Marianne Williamson

Eliminate entertainment pressure. Getting together with friends should be easy and enjoyable. Here are some guidelines for stress-free entertaining:

∗ Shop ahead and prepare ahead.

∗ Choose foods and dishes that require little cooking time.

∗ Don't try recipes for the first time.

Popular action movies are rife with terror and mayhem. Eighty percent of all TV shows portray acts of aggression. This constant barrage of brutality stresses our minds and singes our souls. Instead, watch a comedy or nature show.

Don't go cold turkey. You'll only get discouraged if you try to dump all your couch potato habits at once. Today, trade a half-hour of time-wasting TV for a walk. Or turn off the computer and turn on soft music instead.

With no major investment, you can borrow a treasure from the vast book collection at your local library. Check out books about relaxation, meditation, and exercise.

Do one thing at a time. Time-management experts tell us that to get more done, we should "multitask." But this approach creates pressure and distraction. Instead, focus on one activity at a time. The next time you wash the dinner dishes, pay attention. Wash each one slowly and thoroughly. Completing one task at a time fosters inner serenity as well as true efficiency.

Appreciate the art of lazy days. Sleep late. Stroll to a bakery. Leisurely read the Sunday paper. Go window-shopping. You'll experience a tranquil transformation while you enjoy the most effortless activities.

Ease the transition from work to home. Change into comfortable, casual clothes and leave your work concerns behind.

Make sure to get your share of calming calcium. In addition to building strong bones and teeth, calcium helps regulate healthy nerve and muscle function. A combination of calcium and magnesium acts as a mild relaxant and sleep promoter. Supplemental calcium also relieves premenstrual symptoms.

Take the day off. Remember your joy when school was closed due to bad weather? Don't wait for a storm or a bad cold to take a break. Reward yourself with a Mental Health Day. Cancel all your plans. And don't spend your time trying to catch up. Instead, luxuriate in winding down.

Sea Salt Body Scrub

Try this body scrub to soothe your senses, still your spirit, and smooth your skin.

½ cup fine sea salt
½ cup canola oil
2 tablespoons baking soda
10 drops ylang ylang or Roman chamomile essential oil

1. Combine the sea salt, canola oil, and baking soda, then add the essential oil of your choice and blend well.

2. Moisten your skin with water. Rub small handfuls of the mixture on your arms and legs in circular motions. Wait a few minutes before rinsing.

Cool as a cucumber. Gently place slices of cool cucumber on your closed eyelids. Lie down for 5 minutes. This tension reliever has added visual effects — it temporarily reduces under-eye puffiness.

Don't rush. Remember, life is not a race. Allow yourself time to linger. Relaxation and satisfaction have space to grow only when we slow our pace.

No excuses. Sometimes we mutter, "If I could only get away, I could really relax." We jealously imagine how more fortunate people unwind in style. A famous actress, rich enough to travel to exotic places, revealed her favorite way to relax. She wakes late on a weekend morning and drinks a cup of specialty coffee while reading the *New York Times*. You, too, can create a simple, relaxing weekend ritual.

A good laugh is the "tranquilizer with no side effects." Laughing reduces stress hormone levels, decreases blood pressure, and relieves muscle tension. So yuk it up!

Treat your feet. After being cooped up in shoes all day, these dogs need to dance. Sit in a comfortable chair or lie down.

1. Take off all foot coverings.
2. Alternately flex and extend each foot from the ankle.
3. Make five ankle circles with your right foot.
4. Change directions and do five more.
5. Repeat with your left foot.

Smudging, or burning bundles of sweet-smelling herbs to cleanse odors and energy, is an ancient ritual. To clear the air, light a smudge stick made of sage or cedar. (A stick of incense is an acceptable substitute.) Hold the stick over a shell or a pretty bowl. Walk with it around the room. Waft the fragrant smoke from the floor to the ceiling, then relax in your sacred space.

Imagine an ideal morning. What time would you get out of bed? Who would be the first person to greet you? Would you make time to stretch or jog, write in your journal, or say morning prayers? Would you eat a light breakfast? Use your fantasies to design a graceful awakening.

Lounge in lavender. This fragrant flower is a natural treatment for insomnia, nervousness, and headaches. Lather up with lavender soap or bath gel. If you have a headache, lie down with a lavender-scented compress. Add dried lavender to a cup of herbal tea or punch. And to ensure a restful evening, scent your sheets and pillow with a lavender spray.

On blustery winter nights, hunker down with a hearty stew. Lengthy meal preparation isn't relaxing. Instead, put a few simple ingredients in a pot and let them simmer away.

According to the principles of feng shui, the ancient art of object placement, positioning your bed correctly can improve your sleep as well as your relationships. For optimum health, never put your bed in a direct line with a door or a bathroom. Don't place your bed under beams and don't store items underneath your bed.

Dehydration stresses the body. Drink eight glasses of water every day to help detoxify your blood and eliminate wastes from your body.

Communing with an animal is restorative. The quality of life in nursing homes improves dramatically when pets come to play with the residents. Studies show that stroking a pet helps lower blood pressure. So curl up with a cat or dawdle with a dog.

Go fish. Gather your gear and head outdoors before the rest of the world wakes up. Stop focusing on all the other fish you have to fry and cast away your cares.

Socialize more while preparing less. Invite friends to an old-fashioned potluck. Ask everyone to bring a favorite dish to share. You supply the place, plates, flatware, beverages, and inviting atmosphere.

Keep your camera available and commit to snapping just one still photograph a day. Quiet down to focus while you glimpse life through a lens. Later, reflect as you page through your visual journal.

"There is nothing worth more than this day."

—Johann Wolfgang von Goethe

Squeeze out tension. Try this easy technique to relieve head and neck tension.

1. Place your left palm between your eyebrows and your right palm on the small indentation at the base of your skull.
2. Press and hold for a count of 5.
3. Release, relax for a moment, and then repeat two times.

If vacation travel is not on the horizon, treat yourself to a relaxing afternoon in "another world." Take a solitary trip to a café or bookstore and leave the cellular phone at home.

Delegate or eliminate one 30-minute chore today. Perhaps family members can make their own lunch or do their own laundry. Or alternate shopping or cooking responsibilities with a friend. Be creative — any chore reduction frees up time to relax.

Peppermint Footbath

This footbath will soothe tired feet as it drains stress away.

1 gallon hot water
½ cup dried peppermint OR
4–8 drops peppermint essential oil

1. Fill a basin with steamy water and add either dried peppermint or peppermint essential oil.
2. Sit and submerge.

Beware of stress-causing foods. The additive monosodium glutamate (MSG) can cause headaches and insomnia in sensitive individuals. Limit spicy or fatty foods, especially in the evening, as they can cause heartburn and disturb sleep.

Frolic in the fall foliage. Playing in a pile of autumn leaves is one of the best natural tranquilizers.

A walk in the woods will improve your mood, provide you with a cardiovascular boost, and satisfy you visually. So put on some sturdy boots and grab your day pack to benefit from this great stress reliever.

Don't be the best that you can be. Contrary to popular opinion, trying to be the best at everything doesn't lead to success; it is self-defeating. Perfectionism produces anxiety. Soften your standards on lower-priority items. You will be less frantic when you put your best efforts into activities of greater personal importance.

Communicate from the heart. Clear and concise communication is freeing. Reflect upon what you think, how you feel, and what you want. Then, say what you mean, mean what you say, and don't say it mean.

Beware the ways of the "weekend warrior." Extra chores and active sports on those couple of days off often result in the pains of over-exertion. Soothe away muscle soreness with homeopathic arnica gel found in health food stores and natural pharmacies.

Don't save that exciting bestseller for bedtime — you may not be able to put it down or stop thinking about it once you do. Reserve the half-hour before bed for an unsuspenseful novel or a collection of inspirational short stories.

Spas offer the ultimate relaxation in idyllic settings. Your stay may include meditation, massage, hydrotherapy, yoga, hiking, salon services, and delicious, healthy meals. Or try a day spa as a reasonably priced alternative to full-service programs.